# The

# Ultimate

# Longevity

# Elixir

## The Most Effective

## Life-Extending Natural Beverage

Rory M. Celmin

Editor: Ginny Greene
Cover Design: Rory Celmin

**Contact info:**
email: info@vitalityhealth9.com
website: vitalityhealth9.com
twitter: @VitalityHealth9

ISBN-10: 0-9840186-6-2
ISBN-13: 978-0-9840186-6-6

# ~ <u>Table of Contents</u> ~

# ~ Introduction ~

Could nutrition be the main ingredient to a healthier, longer life? Numerous studies have revealed the effects of nutrition on longevity, and show that the consumption of nutrient-dense foods helps slow the aging process. The American diet today consists mostly of canned, processed, microwave and fast foods which are high in sodium, sugar, white flour, saturated fats and hydrogenated oils which are linked to an increased risk of disease, illness and/or infection. The main factors associated with premature aging are the accumulation of toxins, inflammation and nutritional deficiencies.

What is the best way to obtain all of nature's most healthful foods for disease prevention, improving health and living longer in one serving? The Ultimate Longevity Elixir is the answer. This nutrient-dense, organic beverage has tremendous health benefits. Not only is it vegan and gluten free, it contains no soy, dairy or saturated fat. This elixir combines the most revered culinary ingredients used by cultures/regions that have the highest life expectancy like Asia, the Mediterranean and South America. It was specifically formulated to help eliminate toxins, reduce inflammation, strengthen the immune system, stimulate weight loss, maintain blood sugar and support cardiovascular health in order to slow the aging process. The Ultimate Longevity Elixir helps lower the risk of degenerative disorders, and is the most powerful nutritional solution for enhancing health and increasing longevity.

# ~ <u>List of Ingredients</u> ~

*Apple Cider Vinegar

*Aloe Vera Juice

*Cayenne Pepper

*Garlic

*Ginger

*Lemon

*Turmeric

*Agave

# Apple Cider Vinegar

Apple Cider Vinegar (ACV) is the backbone of the Ultimate Longevity Elixir for several reasons. Approximately 75% of the immune system is located in our stomach, so it is vital to maintain healthy gut bacteria to maximize longevity. Consuming ACV is the equivalent of putting super unleaded fuel in the body. It is actually a 'prebiotic'... so it feeds the healthy microflora (beneficial bacteria) in the stomach and helps strengthen the immune system. It also binds to waste products such as cholesterol, harmful bacteria and toxins and helps eliminate them from the body. ACV is acidic when ingested, but it has an alkaline food ash after digestion so it actually lowers the body's pH and reduces acidity in the body.

*vitamins A, B, C, E, calcium, magnesium, potassium, sulfur, zinc
*stimulates weight loss by breaking down fats/increasing metabolism
*contains *acetic acid* which stops bad (LDL) cholesterol from oxidizing
*reduces effects of food poisoning, bacteria, fungi, viruses, parasites
*lowers triglyceride levels & maintains healthy blood sugar balance
*helps lower cholesterol levels & reduces risk of heart disease
*reduces lactic acid build up helping athletes recover faster
*helps improve memory and protects against dementia
*improves digestive disorders (constipation, IBS)
*improves skin disorders (eczema, psoriasis)
*helps alleviate arthritis and inflammation
*helps ease migraine headaches
*reduces water retention
*anti-cancer properties
*anti-aging properties

# Aloe Vera Juice

Aloe Vera has been used topically to improve skin conditions, as a remedy for sunburns and as a natural moisturizer. When consumed, Aloe Vera juice provides a bounty of health benefits. It is extremely effective for improving numerous digestive disorders (colitis, heartburn, IBS, indigestion), easing arthritis & inflammation and strengthening the immune system. Aloe Vera juice is sugar free, helps maintain healthy blood sugar levels, and contains numerous phytonutrients and amino acids necessary for increased longevity. It has also shown promise in slowing the progression of the AIDS virus by increasing T-4 cell count and lowering P-24 antigen activity.

*vitamins A, B1, B2, B6, B12, C & E, calcium, magnesium & zinc
*helps strengthen immune system & increases white blood cell count
*beneficial for digestive disorders (colitis, heartburn, IBS, indigestion)
*helps alleviate acne, blemishes, burns, cuts, insect stings & infections
*helps improve lung function & protects against lung cancer
*powerful antibacterial, antifungal and antiviral properties
*helps control blood sugar levels and boosts energy
*may help slow the progression of the AIDS virus
*helps increase circulation in the extremities
*helps alleviate arthritis and inflammation
*restores proper pH levels to the body
*detoxifies organs & the bloodstream
*helps reduce hemorrhoids & ulcers
*helps lower cholesterol levels
*promotes cell regeneration
*anti-cancer properties
*anti-aging properties

# Cayenne Pepper

Cayenne pepper has been highly revered for thousands of years for its numerous life-extending health benefits. This red-hot chili pepper is rich in amino acids, and contains a powerful phytonutrient called *capsaicin* that protects DNA from carcinogens, inhibits tumor growth and destroys cancer cells. Cayenne pepper improves cardiovascular health, increases circulation, and helps protect against coronary heart disease. Other benefits of this popular pepper include easing sinus infections, alleviating headaches and migraines, stimulating weight loss by increasing metabolism and improving digestion.

*vitamins B1, B2, B3, B5, B6, C, E & K, calcium
*improving digestion and helping to control flatulence
*stimulates weight loss by increasing metabolism
*helps lowering blood pressure and cholesterol
*alleviating arthritis and inflammation
*alleviating headaches and migraines
*strengthening the immune system
*helps control blood sugar levels
*supports cardiovascular health
*alleviates sinus infections
*inhibits tumor growth
*anti-cancer properties
*anti-aging properties

# Garlic

Garlic is one of the most highly regarded spices that has been effectively used for improving a myriad of health disorders. It contains powerful antioxidants that help reduce the risk of heart attack and stroke, lower blood pressure, improve circulation, detoxify the blood and slow the effects of aging. This highly flavorful bulb impedes the oxidation process of bad (LDL) cholesterol, which helps prevent saturated fats from clogging the arteries and limits oxidative damage to the body. It contains a sulfur compound called *allicin* which inhibits tumor growth, regulates blood sugar and supports liver health. Garlic also helps to alleviate arthritis, strengthens the immune system and protects against colds, fevers & the flu.

*vitamins A, B1, B2, B3, B6, C, calcium, copper, magnesium, manganese, phosphorus, potassium, selenium and zinc
*strengthens the immune system (protects against colds, fevers, flu)
*sulfur compounds bind to heavy metals to remove from body
*thermogenic properties increase body heat & increases metabolism
*contains antibacterial, antiviral & antiparasitic properties
*helps lower cholesterol levels and slows oxidation
*contains *allicin* which helps inhibit tumor growth
*helps maintain healthy blood sugar levels
*helps alleviate arthritis and inflammation
*helps ease asthma and bronchitis
*improves cardiovascular health
*supports healthy liver function
*anti-cancer properties
*anti-aging properties

# Ginger

Ginger is known for its powerful antioxidant properties, and has been used for thousands of years to successfully alleviate various digestive disorders such as motion sickness, nausea, vomiting and diarrhea. It also stimulates circulation, increases blood flow to the extremities, improves cardiovascular health and reduces inflammation essential for increasing longevity. Ginger contains the same blood-thinning quality similar to aspirin that lowers the risk of heart attack or stroke, and protects against colds and the flu by strengthening the immune system. Additionally, it contains a phytonutrient called *zingibain* that is known to dissolve intestinal parasites and their eggs.

*vitamins A, B1, B2, B3, B5, B6, C, E, calcium, iron, magnesium, manganese, phosphorus, potassium, selenium and zinc
*helps relieve joints, muscle cramps, muscle pain and soreness
*antibacterial, antifungal, antiviral, antiparasitic properties
*reduces the risk of arteriosclerosis and atherosclerosis
*effective at relieving a myriad of digestive disorders
*helps maintain healthy blood sugar levels
*helps alleviate arthritis & inflammation
*menstrual discomforts and hot flashes
*helps relieve headaches & migraines
*effective for protecting the liver
*improves cardiovascular health
*helps lower cholesterol levels
*protects against colds and flu
*anti-cancer properties
*anti-aging properties

# Lemon

Lemons are excellent source of vitamin C (ascorbic acid), and contain powerful antioxidant and antibiotic properties. Vitamin C neutralizes free radicals that damage cell membranes, and contain powerful phytonutrients called *flavonoids* that inhibit the growth of cancer cells and help prevent disorders that shorten life. It is known to help prevent heart attacks and strokes, reduce heart disease, repair damaged blood vessels and prevent oxidation of the arteries. Naturally tart and sour, lemons contain antiseptic properties that are effective for both internal and external cleansing. Even though lemons (and limes) are highly acidic upon consumption, they have an alkaline food ash after digestion that helps reduce acidity in the body.

*vitamin C
*helps protect against certain forms of cancer (bladder, lung, skin)
*powerful antiseptic, antioxidant & antibiotic properties
*beneficial for improving asthma & bronchitis
*effective for eliminating intestinal parasites
*lowers risk of cardiovascular disease
*helps remove toxins from the body
*stimulates the immune system
*helps alleviate ear infections
*effective against cholera
*supports kidney health
*anti-cancer properties
*anti-aging properties

# Turmeric

Turmeric is a powerful super-spice that been used in western India since 600 BC as flavoring, as a dye, and as medicine. It is one of the most powerful antioxidants, and has been very effective for alleviating arthritis, inflammation and combating diabetes. Turmeric has been used to help reduce the risk of leukemia as well as colon, breast, lung, ovarian, pancreatic, prostate, stomach & skin cancer. Its active ingredient, *curcumin,* is responsible for the yellowish color of curry and mustards and is associated with increased longevity. Turmeric has also shown promise in combating Alzheimer's disease, as it helps break up beta-amyloid plaques collected in the brain. Elderly people of India rarely develop dementia, which is believed to be related to the regular consumption of turmeric.

*vitamins B1, B2, B3 & C, calcium, potassium and zinc
*extremely effective for alleviating arthritis & inflammation
*lowers cholesterol levels & reduces risk of heart disease
*increases blood circulation & normalizes blood sugar
*detoxifies the liver & helps regenerate liver tissue
*reduces risk of developing polyps in the colon
*lowers risk of cardiovascular disease
*alleviates effects of food poisoning
*helps eliminate intestinal parasites
*strengthens the immune system
*improves asthma & bronchitis
*helps relieve cystic fibrosis
*improves intestinal flora
*anti-cancer properties
*anti-aging properties

# Agave

Agave (raw) is a nutritious, natural 'vegan' sweetener that contains fructose, but has a low glycemic-index score so it is much healthier that refined sugar and is a much better option for those with diabetes. It contains a class of phytonutrients called *saponins* which help reduce inflammation and lower cholesterol levels. Agave also contains powerful anti-aging properties that synthesize hyaluronic acid, which hydrates the skin and helps prevent wrinkles. The sweetness of agave balances out the Ultimate Longevity Elixir, and provides many important health benefits.

*dietary fiber, calcium, iron and zinc
*contains *inulin* that provides beneficial bacteria for the stomach
*lowers bad (LDL) cholesterol & triglyceride levels
*contains *saponins* which reduces inflammation
*helps hydrate skin & reduce wrinkles
*inhibits cholesterol absorption
*reduces risk of constipation
*inhibits tumor growth
*anti-cancer properties
*anti-aging properties

# ~ <u>Ingredients</u> ~

1 cup – apple cider vinegar

1 cup – aloe vera juice

1/8 tsp – cayenne pepper

2 grams – garlic (crushed)

1 oz – fresh ginger (peeled)

1 – lemon (juice of)

3 tbsp – turmeric (powder)

2 tbsp – agave (raw)

+

2 cups – water

Makes approx. 32 fluid ounces

# ~ <u>Preparation</u> ~

**Step 1:** Add agave to water (room temperature) to dissolve

**Step 2:** Add turmeric and cayenne pepper to agave/water solution, stir well until both are thoroughly mixed

**Step 3:** In a blender, combine agave/water/cayenne/turmeric mix, apple cider vinegar, garlic, ginger and fresh lemon juice

**Step 4:** Blend thoroughly for about 10-20 seconds, or until ginger pieces are mostly dissolved

**Step 5:** Add aloe vera juice and blend for an additional 5-10 seconds

**Step 6:** Serve over ice or drink as a shot, store remaining elixir in glass bottles or containers in the refrigerator.

*increase or decrease amount of agave to alter sweetness*

Enjoy the most healthful, life-extending elixir ever created! Sip first thing in the morning for a detox cleanse and energy boost, drink after meals to ease heartburn or indigestion, or once a day as preventive maintenance to maximize health. Here's a toast to your new-found energy, feeling of well-being and enhanced longevity. *Cheers!*

# ~ List of References ~

*Anderson, Jean E. M.S., Deskins, Barbara Ph.D. *The Nutrition Bible – A Comprehensive No-Nonsense Guide to Foods, Nutrients, Additives, Preservatives, Pollutants and Everything Else We Eat and Drink.* New York, NY: HarperCollins Publishers, 1997

*Balch, Phyllis A., CNC. *Prescription for Nutritional Healing, 5th edition.* New York, NY: Penguin Group (Avery), 2010

*Beck, Leslie R.D. *Leslie Beck's Nutrition Encyclopedia.* Toronto, Ontario: Penguin Group, 2003

*Campbell, T. Colin, Ph.D., and Campbell, Thomas M. *The China Study – Startling Implications for Diet, Weight Loss and Long-term Health.* Dallas, TX: BenBella Books, 2005

*Colbert, Don M.D. *Toxic Relief – Restore Health and Energy Through Fasting and Detoxification.* Lake Mary, FL: Siloam Press, 2003

*Miller, David Niven. *Grow Youthful – A Practical Guide to Slowing Your Aging.* Cottesloe, West Australia: John Hunt Publishing & O-Books, 2007

*Murray, Michael N.D. and Pizzorno, Joseph N.D. with Pizzorno, Lara M.A., L.M.T. *The Encyclopedia of Healing Foods.* New York, NY: Atria Books, 2005

*Plasker, Eric D.C. *The 100 Year Lifestyle.* Avon, MA: Adams Media Publishing, 2007

*Price, Weston A., D.D.S. *Nutrition and Physical Degeneration, 8th edition.* San Diego, CA: Price-Pottenger Nutrition Foundation, 2008

*Roizen, Michael F., M.D. and Oz, Mehmet C., M.D. *You Staying Young – The Owners Manual for Extending Your Warranty.* New York, NY: Free Press, 2007

*Tessmer, Kimberly A. R.D., L.D. *The Everything Nutrition Book – Boost Energy, Prevent Illness and Live Longer.* Avon, MA: Adams Media, 2003

*Trattler, Ross N.D., D.O. and Jones, Adrian N.D. *Better Health Through Natural Healing, 2nd edition.* Heatherton VIC, Australia: Hinkler Books, 2001

*Trowell, Hubert C. and Burkitt, Denis P. *Western Diseases: Their Emergence and Prevention.* Cambridge, MA: Harvard University Press, 1981

*Wilson, Dr. Lawrence. *Legal Guidelines for Unlicensed Practitioners.* Prescott, AZ: L.D. Wilson Consultants, 2007

*Yeager, Selene. *The Doctor's Book of Food Remedies.* Emmaus, PA: Rodale Press Inc., 2000

# ~ <u>Nutrition Glossary</u> ~

## A

**Absorption** – the process of assimilating nutrients into the body

**Adaptogen** – herbal substances that reduce stress and produce beneficial adjustments in the body

**Alpha-carotene** – a phytonutrient found in carrots that is beneficial for eye health

**Alpha-linolenic acid** (ALA) – omega-3 essential fatty acid found in flaxseed, pumpkin & soybean oils

**Amino acid** – nitrogen and carbon-based organic compounds that build protein and muscle

**Anabolic** – substance that helps convert nutrition into building and repairing muscle tissues in the body

**Antacid** – a substance that neutralizes stomach acid

**Antibody** – immune system protein that combats bacteria, fungus and other foreign substances

**Antigen** – a substance that provokes the creation of antibodies

**Antihistamine** – a substance that binds with histamine receptors and reduces the effects of histamines

**Antioxidant** – a substance that minimizes free radical damage to the heart, arteries, and tissues, such as vitamins, minerals and nutrients

**Arachidonic acid** (AA) – an omega-6 essential fatty acid found in eggs, meat, poultry and shellfish

**Ascorbic acid** – the organic compound known as vitamin C

# B

**Beta carotene** – phytonutrient with antioxidant properties the body uses to produce vitamin A, found in broccoli, carrots, collard greens, kale, pumpkin, spinach and sweet potatoes

**Bio-availability** – the ease of which nutrients can be absorbed into the body

**Bioflavonoid** – a group of active substances essential for the absorption of vitamin C

**Blood sugar** – concentration of glucose in the blood

# C

**Carbohydrate** – organic substances that are our the main source of energy in our diets

**Carcinogen** – a toxic substance capable of producing cancer

**Carotene** – a substance that is converted into vitamin A in the body

**Cartenoids** – phytonutrients that contain antioxidant properties

**Cellulose** – an organic carbohydrate from fruits and vegetables

**Chelation** – chemical process where molecules bind to a mineral atom increasing its bio-availability

**Chelation therapy** – the introduction of substances into the body to remove heavy metals

**Chlorophyll** – the green pigment in plants that is vital for photosynthesis; converting light into energy

**Cholesterol** – steroid metabolite compound including lipids (fats) naturally produced by the body, a structural component of cell membranes, helps absorption of fatty acids; HDL (good) and LDL (bad)

**Citric acid** – organic acid found in citrus fruits

**Coenzyme** – a substance that works with enzymes to promote normal enzyme activity

**Complete protein** – a protein that contains all 8 essential amino acids

**Complex carbohydrate** – a carbohydrate that provides fiber and slowly releases sugar into the body

**Conjugated Linoleic Acid** (CLA) – a naturally occurring fatty-acid that helps reduce body fat

**Cordyceps** – rare medicinal mushroom used in Traditional Chinese Medicine for over 5,000 years to strengthen the immune system, improve adrenal function, lower blood pressure and cholesterol, prevent kidney disease and liver disorders

**Cortisol** – one of the main catabolic hormones in the body

**Creatine** – a high-energy compound in muscle cells which stores energy and increases strength

**Cruciferous** – 'cross-shaped' blossoms that support digestive health (broccoli, cabbage, cauliflower)

**D**

**Detoxification** – process of eliminating toxic substances from the body

**Diuretic** – substance that increases urine flow

**Docosahexaenoic acid** (DHA) – an omega-3 essential fatty acid found in marine micro-algae, anchovies, cod, mackerel, salmon and tuna

**E**

**Eicosapentaenoic acid** (EPA) – an omega-3 essential fatty acid found in cod, salmon, sardines and tuna

**Electrolytes (**potassium, sodium and chloride) – soluble substances containing free ions that are capable of conducting electric impulses throughout the body

**Enzyme –** a protein catalyst that manages or increases chemical reactions in the body

**Essential Fatty Acids** (EFA's) – amino acids that cannot be synthesized by the body and must be supplied by foods or supplements

**F**

**Fat-soluble** – the ability to dissolve in fats and oils

**Fatty acid –** a carboxylic acid derived from natural fats and oils

**Fiber –** indigestible plant matter that helps eliminate toxins from the body (fruits, vegetables, nuts, legumes, whole grains)

**Flavonoid –** a class of metabolite substances found in plants that help protect against cancer

**Fructose – a** sugar found in fruit that has a low glycemic index

**G**

**Gamma-linolenic acid** (GLA) – an omega-6 essential fatty acid found in borage & primrose oil

**Gland –** an organ that synthesizes substances for release into the bloodstream

**Glucose –** a simple sugar in the blood that is the major energy source for the body's cells and functions

**Gluten –** a protein found in oats, wheat, barley and rye

**Glycemic Index** (GI) – measure of how much food raises blood sugar levels as compared to white bread, which has a GI of 100 (the lower the number the less insulin is released by the body)

**Glycogen** – the main form of glucose stored in the body, then converts back to glucose to supply energy

**Growth Hormone** (GH) – a hormone that is released by the pituitary gland that promotes muscle growth and the breakdown of body fat for energy, subsides with age

# H

**HDL cholesterol** (high-density lipoprotein) – known as *good cholesterol*, it helps clear fat from the bloodstream and indicates a low risk of cardiovascular disease

**Heavy metals** (arsenic, cadmium, lead, mercury) – elements that possess metallic properties and have a gravity measurement greater than 5.0

**Herbal therapy** – herbal combination of tincture extracts and capsules used for cleansing and healing

**Histamine** – chemical released by the immune system that has potential negative effects on the body

**Homeopathy** – alternative medicines using herbs, natural substances to strengthen the immune system

**Hormone** – vital substances produced by the body that regulates many biological processes

**Hydrochloric acid** (HCL) – a strong corrosive stomach acid that helps digestion

**Hydrogenation** – process by which hydrogen atoms are combined with oil molecules to turn liquid oils into solids, destroying the nutritional value of the oil

**Hypoallergenic** – having a low capacity for being affected by allergies

# I

**Immune system** – a complex system of organs, cells and proteins that protect the body against disease

**Inorganic** – substances that do not contain carbon

**Insulin** – an anabolic hormone produced by the pancreas that regulates proper blood sugar levels

**Intestinal flora** – friendly bacteria in the digestive tract that are essential for digestion and metabolism

**Isoflavones** – a class of phytonutrients that protect against estrogen-based cancers like breast cancer

# K

**Kefir** – fermented milk product that contains anti-aging properties

**Ketosis** – a process of metabolism where the liver converts fats into fatty acids and is used for energy

**Kombucha** – a sweetened fermented tea beverage that has detoxifying effects and healing properties

# L

**Lactase** – an enzyme that converts lactose into glucose and is necessary for digesting milk and dairy

**Lactic acid** – an acid created from glucose metabolism that accumulates in the body after strenuous exercise causing muscle fatigue and pain

**Lactose** – term referring to milk sugar

**Lauric acid** – a fatty acid found in coconut and palm kernel oil that has antimicrobial properties

**LDL cholesterol** (low density lipoprotein) – known as *bad cholesterol* that may cause cardiovascular disease

**Legumes** – seed pod that splits both sides when ripe (alfalfa, beans, carob, lentils, peanuts, peas, soy)

**Lentils** – a leguminous, climbing-vine plant containing only 2 seeds to a pod (beluga, black, green, red, white, yellow)

**Liminoids** – phytonutrients found in citrus fruits that help inhibit the production of cancer cells and HIV protease activity

**Linolenic acid** (LA) – an omega-6 essential fatty acid found in corn oil, safflower and sunflower oil

**Lipids** – natural substances that are soluble in the same solvents as fats and oils

**Lipolysis** – refers to the chemical breakdown of body fat by enzymes that produce energy

**Lipoprotein** – protein molecule that helps transport fats around the bloodstream

**Lipotropic** – substances that help break down fat during metabolism and manage blood sugar levels

**Lutein** – phytonutrient that helps protect against macular degeneration (spinach, kale, turnip greens)

**Lycopene** – a phytonutrient that helps protect against prostate cancer and ultraviolet rays from the sun found in guava, pink grapefruit, tomatoes and watermelon

# M

**Macrobiotics** – referring to a branch of Eastern medicine that uses grain as a staple food, and balances Yin (negative) and Yang (positive) foods together to overcome health issues

**Macronutrients** (proteins, carbohydrates and fats) – essential elements needed in large quantities to sustain proper health

**Malabsorption** – the inability to absorb nutrients from the intestines into the bloodstream

**Metabolism** – process by which cells absorb nutrition and change food into energy

**Mineral** – naturally occurring substance that is essential for human life and vital to metabolic processes

**Monounsaturated fats** (canola, olive, peanut and sunflower oils) – fatty acids that are not saturated with hydrogen, typically liquid at room temperature but will solidify when refrigerated

# N

**Naturopathy** – alternative form of medicine using a combination of natural methods to combat disease and maintain health

**Nonessential Amino Acids** – amino acids that can be produced by the body from other amino acids, therefore not essential to the human diet

**Nutrient** – a natural substance that all living organisms need for growth and survival

**Nutrition** – the science of turning food into fuel for the body to use

# O

**Organic** – referring to foods that are grown naturally, without the use of synthetic chemicals like herbicides, pesticides or hormones

**Oxalates** (oxalic acid) – organic substances found in humans, plants and animals of which high concentrations may lead to kidney stones; (oxalic acid foods include: amaranth, beans, beet greens, beer, berries, celery, chocolate, figs, kale, kiwi, leeks, nuts/seeds, okra, parsley, plums, quinoa, rhubarb, soy foods, spinach, squash, Swiss chard, tangerines, watercress, wheat germ)

# P

**Parasite** – a smaller organism living on/inside of a larger host, it is completely dependent on its host for nourishment and can be potentially damaging

**Pepsin** – a digestive enzyme released by the stomach to break down food proteins into peptides

**Peptide** – a compound made up of two or more amino acids that are broken down by protein molecules

**pH** (potential of hydrogen) – a measurement of the acidity and alkalinity of a substance or solution

**Photosynthesis** – the synthesis of organic compounds from inorganic compounds by plants and algae involving light energy

**Phytonutrients** – natural substances found in fruits and vegetables that protect the body against disease (chlorophyll, carotenoids, flavonoids, isoflavones, inositol, lignans, indoles, phenols, sulfides, terpenes)

**Polyphenols** – a group of compounds found in plants that have at least one phenol unit per molecule

**Polysaccharides** – a class of carbohydrates which breaks down during hydrolysis to a monosaccharide

**Probiotics** – substances that promote the growth of friendly bacteria in the body

**Protein** – nitrogen-based organic compounds made from amino acids that are the basic components of animal and vegetable tissues, needed for growth and repair

**Proteolytic enzymes** – enzymes that break down proteins and reduce the risk of cancer

**Purines** – natural substances that are part of the chemical structure of human, plant and animal genes, high concentrations may lead to arthritis, gout and inflammation (purine-rich foods include: anchovies, asparagus, bacon, beef, cauliflower, chicken, eggs, ham, herring, mackerel, mushrooms, mussels, oatmeal, organ meats, peas, pork, sardines, shellfish, smelt, spinach, sweetbreads, turkey, yeast),

# R

**RDA** (Recommended Daily Allowance) – the basic amount of nutrients that should be consumed daily to maintain proper health

**Retinoic acid** – the acid from vitamin A

# S

**Saliva** – a mixture of water, protein and salts that makes food easy to swallow and digest

**Saturated fat** (butter, chocolate, dairy, lard, meat) – regarded as unhealthy fat, it is typically solid at room temperature and has been shown to raise cholesterol levels

**Simple carbohydrate** – a carbohydrate that is quickly digested and absorbed into the bloodstream

**Stevia** – a natural herbal sweetener native to South America that is much sweeter than sugar

**Sucrose** – table sugar

**Synergy** – the harmonious interaction between two or more substances where their combined ability is greater than their individual actions

## T

**Thermogenics** – dietary supplements that increase metabolism and generate heat

**Thyroid gland** – internal thermostat regulating body temperature by secreting hormones that control energy used and calories burned

**Tolerance** – the capability of an organism to endure an unfavorable environment

**Toxin** – a poison that impairs health and bodily functions

**Trace element** – mineral required by the body in minute quantities for proper growth and development

**Trans-fat** – unsaturated fat produced through hydrogenation; increases risk of cardiovascular disease

**Triglyceride** – compound made up of three fatty acids and glycerol and is how fat is stored in the body

## U

**Unsaturated fat** (olive, flaxseed, safflower and fish oils) – known as healthy fat, these help reduce cholesterol and triglycerides levels in the blood

## V

**Vitamin** – organic substance obtained through diet to maintain proper health and support many biological functions

## W

**Water-soluble** – the ability to dissolve in water

# X

**Xylitol** – a natural sweetener made from birch bark that has antifungal properties, has a low glycemic index (GI) score and alkalizes the body

# Y

**Yang** (heat, light and dryness) – one of two essential principles of Chinese medicine needed to create balance and harmony in the body, organs include the gallbladder, spleen, intestines and skin

**Yin** (cold, shadow and moisture) – the other essential principle of Chinese medicine needed to create balance and harmony in the body, organs include the liver, heart, kidneys, lungs and bones

# Z

**Zeaxanthin** – a phytonutrient that protects against macular degeneration found in citrus fruits, eggs and green vegetables

# ~ <u>About the Author</u> ~

Rory M. Celmin is certified in sports nutrition from the International Fitness Professional Association (IFPA), received a Bachelor's Degree in English from California State University San Marcos (CSUSM) and has studied health and nutrition for over 25 years. He is the author of *Nature's Nutrition – A Comprehensive Resource Guide for Super Foods, Natural Supplements and Preventative Health* and *Top 25 Nutritional Health Supplements,* and also offers personalized nutritional consulting online at Vitality Health Solutions (vitalityhealth9.com). In his spare time he enjoys basketball, tennis, surfing, hiking and photography, and resides in sunny California.

**Website:** vitalityhealth9.com
**Contact:** info@vitalityhealth9.com
**Facebook:** Vitality Health Solutions
**Instagram:** vitality_health_solutions
**Twitter:** @VitalityHealth9